COLOUR, HEALING AND THE HUMAN SOUL

Understanding colours and using them for health and therapy

Gladys Mayer

GW00538316

RUDOLF STEINER PRESS

Rudolf Steiner Press
Hillside House, The Square
Forest Row, East Sussex RH18 5ES

www.rudolfsteinerpress.com

This edition published by Rudolf Steiner Press 2019

First published as two separate booklets: *Colour and the Human Soul*
(1954) and *Colour and Healing* (1960) by New Knowledge Books

A catalogue record for this book is available from the British Library

ISBN 978 1 85584 565 7

Cover by Andrew Morgan Design
Typeset by Vman InfoTech, Chennai, India
Printed and bound by 4Edge Ltd., Essex

CONTENTS

PUBLISHER'S NOTE

This little book was written by one of the pioneers of Rudolf Steiner's work in Great Britain. It was originally published as two separate booklets: *Colour and the Human Soul* in 1954 and *Colour and Healing* in 1960. Whilst the bulk of the content remains relevant to the present time, some outer aspects of the text reflect the context in which it was written, and will thus appear dated. Nevertheless, we consider that the book contains many original insights and ideas, and trust that readers will continue to find it of value.

PART ONE

COLOUR AND THE HUMAN SOUL

What is colour? – fleeting, insubstantial fluctuating; always changing, yet in itself ever the same. Colour is a mystery if we try to understand it in physical terms.

What is it that holds colour to substance, what releases it? Colour is always the same in itself; green is green whenever we meet it; yellow is yellow. But when attached to substance, the green of today may be yellow tomorrow, and yellow turns to red, to brown, to grey—the colour of decay. Colour attaches itself to substance in the natural world but so lightly is it attached that it may change from minute to minute, from hour to hour. It arises in one place and fades away in another. It is held fast for years, as in the minerals, or it changes from day to day, as in the plants. Colour attached to the natural world is transient, fluctuating, changeful, playing as it were over the substance rather than deeply embodied. Yet in itself it is unchanging, timeless.

A glimpse into the nature and origin of colour may be gained by considering the splendour of colour in the sky at dawn or at sunset, or again the ethereal beauty of the rainbow glowing against a grey, stormy sky. Why is it that sunrise and sunset paint the sky with wondrous colours in a way the pure radiance of the midday sun fails to do? Why is it that the rainbow appears clearest against a lowering sky?

Goethe's theory of colour gives the answer to this problem in a way that corresponds with artistic feeling and experience. Modern physics gives another explanation which does not in the least correspond with artistic experience but may have significance in other spheres. Goethe's theory has been set aside by the physicists, but Rudolf Steiner not only shows experimentally that it is well founded in reality but he also shows historically how in Goethe there was reborn an ancient spiritual wisdom concerning the nature of colour, of which Aristotle had preserved a last remnant, but which, between the times of Aristotle and Goethe, had been utterly lost.

This ancient wisdom taught that colour, both in the outer world and in the inner life of the soul, arises through the mingling of darkness and of light. Colour, according to this teaching, is not merely split-up components of light but it is an active mingling of the forces of darkness and of light. Darkness in this case is not, as in modern physics, a mere absence of light, but is *in itself an actuality*. Light and darkness meet and interact and from their interaction colour arises.

As Goethe puts it: 'Colours are the deeds and sufferings of the light'. What it suffers is from darkness. Hence the sunrise colours, driving away darkness and the colours of sunset, when darkness draws near.

By Rudolf Steiner's teaching of anthroposophy we are led still further into the mystery of colour and begin to understand not only the nature and origin of colour, but its significance for ourselves. What is the significance of colour? Is it merely a matter of like and dislike? This colour is sympathetic to me, and that colour antipathetic. Is it purely a matter of subjective feeling, or is it something more?

Anthroposophy shows us that colour is, as it were, the breath of life to the soul. We not only live our feeling life in colour, but in fact, as Rudolf Steiner puts it, the ego is colour. We live inwardly so entirely in colour as to be indistinguishable from colour itself. Colour is the real garment of the spiritual being whose outermost covering is the human physical body. Colour is the visible element in which the invisible makes itself evident. Throughout the whole of the physical world the same thing is true—spirit radiant in matter takes colour as its most subtle and intimate manifestation.

6

Colour is to the spiritual life what food and air and water are to the physical life. As these nourish our bodies, so colour nourishes the soul and spirit.

Rudolf Steiner pictures for us the Earth breathing its soul in and out in weaving colours; breathing in the colours radiated to it from the stars, breathing them out again in the coloured astral life of souls on Earth. Colour is the gift of the planets to the Earth, caught and held fast in the minerals, fleetingly in the plants and flowers which are like the mirrored reflection of the stars.

In the life of man, colour is breathed in and out continually, albeit unconsciously. In waking life, colour is, as it were, breathed in through the sense of sight and brings quickening and healing powers to the spirit. And in sleep, man's spiritual and astral being is breathed in colour out of his sleeping physical body to expand to the world of stars—i.e., the astral world of colour. And to clairvoyant consciousness the form of his astral being is just colour—weaving, changeful, glowing, transparent colours.

Picture what has happened. In ancient times the spirit of man, living under divine-spiritual guidance, inspired by breathing in the substance of divine wisdom, living as the child of God incapable of evil, came down to Earth from spiritual heights, clad in a wondrous garment of rainbow-coloured light, the gift of the stars from whence it came. On Earth man became loosed from divine guidance, he attained individuality and freedom, freedom to learn to love, and freedom to fall into error. The cosmic harmonies, rhythms and colours in his being were disturbed; disharmony, uncertainty, disorder and impurity came in. The picture of how far that disturbance has gone can be obtained in every free and spontaneous individual creation in a work of art of child or student or artist, for art gives a living picture not only of the soul of its creator but also of the soul-condition of the world in which he lives, of the soul of his race, of his epoch. As the artist progresses, his pictures become less and less pictures of his own soul and more and more the mirror of the World-Soul. But in all cases they reflect, as in a mirror, this life in colour which man inherits from the stars but into which disorder has crept.

But now, through consciousness, through art, man can, out of his own free spirit, begin to take the cosmic laws and harmonies into his being. He can begin to recreate divine harmony in the Earth-being through his own free act. This is art in its essence: to seek to understand and recreate the divine harmonies in earthly substance, to bring light into darkness, to weave the divine and the earthly together into a new, colourful harmony.

How is he to do this?

Again let us turn to Goethe and Newton and compare their views regarding the world of colour, both of them were characteristic of the men who put them forth.

Newton, inspired by the scientific, analytical spirit of his age, made his theory of colour as split up light by looking at the rays of sunlight coming through a narrow slit in a shuttered window; he narrowed his field of vision, as it were.

Goethe, the poet, approaching his science from the artist's feeling for the unity of the whole of life, approaching it in the universal sense, came to quite different conclusions about light and darkness. He widened his field of vision and obtained different results. His view of colour as the interweaving of light and darkness is the result.

What can happen to our colour-sense if we look at it out of the narrow slit of personal taste, of personality? The small errors and disturbances of our own life of soul, of our own unregulated astral bodies, may well continue to make our cosmic colour-sense muddy and unclear. But if we expand our colour perception beyond the sphere of sympathies and antipathies to the understanding of colour in its real nature, we begin to bring the essence of colour-harmony into our own being, into our life of feeling.

To gain this understanding of the colour in a quite real and living form, it is essential to enter more fully and consciously than is usual both into the experience our senses give us of the physical world as it lies before us—a creation of forms, movement and colour—and again into the inner world of imagination which lives for nearly everyone in the experience of dreams, with their rapidly changing forms and wonderful glowing colours freed from substantial content.

For the artist, colour is a pathway to experience of a non-substantial world, of a realm of spiritual reality which is the real origin both of the substantial forms of the physical world perceptible to our senses, and of the insubstantial forms which flit arbitrarily and elusively through our dream-consciousness, or which are built consciously, following a law of inner necessity, into creative works of art.

To understand the laws governing artistic creation we do not turn to the physical world and faithfully copy it, as has been the trend of past art, but rather we try to perceive behind the sense-perceptible forms that which has not yet found expression, that which the physical world is striving to produce, which it has not yet produced and can only produce through the instrument of human intelligence—i.e., of the spirit working in human consciousness.

If, for example, we look at a growing plant, we perceive, through our senses, the plant in its then stage of growth; but with imagination or even through the faculty of memory, we may recall the plant as it was in its first stages of growth, how the first green shoots pushed themselves forth from the dark Earth, and as we recall this and the later stages leading to the plant as we see it now, we begin to realize that what in reality is revealed to the senses in the plant is only a kind of image of a living moment, a process of growth, expansion, metamorphosis, which never really ceases for an instant, but which our ordinary senses are not able to perceive. This indeed is the reality in the plant-world which nature unfolds before us in a series of images succeeding one another in time. Imaginative vision can lay hold of the process itself and so come nearer to the source of living creation.

To understand colour in a similar way is more difficult, for colour is indeed an experience of the soul which may so far differ individually as to appear to have a very uncertain foundation in objective reality. It is precisely because of this insubstantiality in colour that it may become the greatest aid to us in passing from the sense-perceptible world to experience gained beyond ordinary sense-perceptions.

Following the same method as previously indicated, we may follow the experience of light coming into darkness—i.e., a sunrise—either imaginatively or in the physical world. We can imagine the whole dark sky above us, grey before the dawn, transforming itself to bluish colour as the light begins to ray across it. We can see the pale golden gleams of light breaking the horizon while the rosy pinks and mauves above bring life and colour into the sombre blue; and then the whole power and vivid orange-red-gold glory of the sun breaking through shrouding mists and lighting up the cold darkness of the Earth. We can watch the process happening in nature and re-create it in memory, or we may create the process by inner imagination. In either case we begin to enter livingly into the source of colour.

Colour arises through the interweaving of light and darkness. What is perceptible in the physical world as a sense-experience— i.e., colour arising when light flows into darkness, may also be perceived in the inner life of the soul as a law of its own nature. Colour, in the life of the soul, becomes possible only when light flows into darkness, or darkness into light.

The rhythm and balance of feeling, working between the light of conscious thinking and the dark unconscious forces of will, displays itself in the soul's life, in colour. Were we beings of *thought* only, a cold clear light irradiating all would be characteristic of our inner life; were we beings of *will* only, the soul would express itself in turgid darkness.

But between the two extremes, the feeling soul expresses itself in warmth and colour in the imaginative creations of art. In this sphere of imaginative creation, the soul can work out the spiritual laws of the cosmic, universal harmonies, give them again as a kind of echo of the immeasurably great and majestic forms, rhythms and harmonies of the world of sun and stars. The soul can do this consciously, because the same laws are living in our being as guide the sun and stars. Night after night when the narrowed consciousness of day-experience closes with our closed eyelids, the human soul-and-spirit expands towards the world of planets, sun, moon and the fixed stars, experiencing these like a part of its own being, so that it is no unknown process that we have to conjure up when we seek the universal harmonies, but it is a reality experienced and contained secretly within our own being. To the imaginative consciousness, colour is a way of regaining that experience consciously.

In one of the series of lectures on the Gospel of St Luke, Rudolf Steiner gives a clear description of how it is possible to rise to an understanding of the imaginative world by the pathway of colour, starting from the visible world. He says that the imaginative world is formed in such a way that we may gain an idea of it by picturing a plant before us, from which we are able to draw forth everything perceptible to the sense of sight as 'colour', so that it floats as a mere form—freely in the air. If we were to do no more than draw forth the colours from the plant, we should have a lifeless colour form before us. But to the clairvoyant this colour form does not remain a lifeless colour picture at all, for when he draws forth from the object what is within it as colour, then, through the preparation he has undergone, this colour picture begins to be animated by spirit, just as in the sense-world the plants are animated by matter. He then has before him, not a lifeless colour form, but coloured light, floating freely, changing colour, and flashing in the most diverse ways, full of inward life, so that each colour is the expression of the peculiarity of a being of soul-and-spirit imperceptible to the sense-world: that is, to the clairvoyant, the colour in the material plant becomes the expression of beings of soul-and-spirit.

Now imagine a world filled with these colour forms, reflecting in the most diverse ways, continually changing and altering their shapes, your vision not confined to the colours as in a painting of glimmering colour-reflections—but imagine it all as the expression of being of soul-and-spirit, so that we may say to ourselves: 'When a green colour picture flashes up, it is to me the expression of something intellectual behind it; or when a clear red colour flashes up, it is to me the expression of a passionate being.' Now imagine this whole sea of interlacing colours—we might equally use another picture and say a mass of interacting perceptions, or perceptions of taste or of smell, for all these are the expressions of beings of soul-and-spirit standing behind them—and we have what is called the 'Imaginative' world. It is nothing to which we can apply the word 'imagination' in its ordinary usage; it is not a fancy—it is a real world. It is a different mode of comprehension from that of the senses.

Within this Imaginative world we encounter everything that lies behind the sense-world, yet not perceptible to the physical senses.

If we can rise to an understanding of this living world of colour, this 'Imaginative World' as Rudolf Steiner described it, so that we can feel its reality, how does this throw light on the problem of colour for us, and on the living in colour which is the path of art to spiritual consciousness?

In pictures experienced between sleeping and waking, and in those dreams which carry us out of the physical world into a more vivid and colourful experience than sense-life has ever known, we have already a hint of this world of colour which stands behind the dream. But it is an elusive, fleeting phantom of a world, vanishing almost as soon as it is experienced, and one from which we can only rarely carry anything of value clearly forth.

Quite other is the experience if with fully awakened day-consciousness we seek deliberately to enter into the life of colour and unite ourselves with it, so that we can to some extent at least experience what Rudolf Steiner described as the clairvoyant's experience of the Imaginative world.

BLUE

For example, we can sink ourselves into a single colour and unite ourselves with it. If we unite ourselves with the colour blue, for example, we can begin to feel its cosmic quality, to feel how it carried us away beyond the experience of our own enclosed ego to the experience of the infinite, of devotion, of self-surrender. We can feel about blue as we feel when we gaze into the dark, unfathomable blue of heaven in a clear midday sky, as though the immeasurable spaces of a mighty universe surround us, shield us, cover us; and whilst the blueness draws us out of ourselves into infinite distance, at the same time something not only comforting but tenderly forming us, sheltering and shaping our inner life, giving it boundaries and form, appears to stream back to us from the blue. It is as though the soul were being lured to infinite distance only at last to find itself in a greater reality. Goethe says of blue: 'This colour has a curious and unutterable effect for the eye. It is, as colour, a force. But it stands on the negative side, and is in its greatest purity as it were a charming nothingness. It has in appearance something contradictory, of stimulant and of rest.'

Rudolf Steiner says of the colour blue that if we could enter wholly into its mood of self-surrender and devotion and remain in it sufficiently long, there would come a feeling at last of being blessed by divine mercy, by divine compassion.

As regards the painting of blue, in his three lectures on colour, Rudolf Steiner speaks of what lies in the nature of the colour itself and how it asks to be painted. One always feels that, to him, colour is a living entity, the outer manifestation of a living, spiritual being, and that we are therefore in a way imprisoning this spiritual being if we merely lay a colour between outlines in a preconceived pattern, or according to any already thought-out plan or design. For thought is essentially an after-copy of spiritual intelligence or spiritual creative imagination out of which real art springs.

Hence, for art to follow after thought is to make the living follow the dead, or to imprison living, creative impulse with unlimited possibilities of expansion and growth, within a restricted, hardened concept of the physical brain which no longer has any possibility of expansion, but is, as it were, the cast-off corpse of a living, spiritual truth.

And so in the matter of colour, it is of no value merely to collect intellectual concepts. Each of these concepts must become a matter of living *experience* through individual effort. In the sphere of art, one can only create out of real experience, not out of any lightly accepted theory, and until one has made this experience one's own it is unproductive.

What a poet says of truth applies very fully in this sphere to the experience of colour, or indeed to all experience of the spiritual worlds:

> Many loved Truth, and lavished life's best oil
> Amid the dust of books to find her,
> Content at last as guerdon of their toil
> With the cast mantle she has left behind her.
> Many in sad faith sought for her,
> Many with crossed hands sighed for her,
> But these our brothers fought for her,
> At life's dear peril wrought for her –
> So loved her that they died for her,
> Tasting the raptured sweetness
> Of her divine completeness.

GREEN AND RED

In the same way as we have endeavoured to penetrate into the mood of blue, we may now attempt to come into relation with other colours.

Before us lies the whole rainbow-scale of colours: violet, dark blue, light blue, green, yellow, orange, red—each with its own character, its own life and quality. On the one side the colours where light predominates—red, orange, yellow; on the other side the colours where dark predominates—blue, indigo, violet; and between, the neutral mixture, green.

Rudolf Steiner adds yet another colour to the scale visible in prismatic experiments, which he, in accord with Goethe, calls 'peach-blossom' colour. This colour, which is of particular interest, will be discussed later. Let us confine ourselves at present to the scale of seven colours in their physical appearance.

According to Goethe, blue arises when darkness is seen through light, as e.g., the blue sky, space darkness seen through sunlight, or a window pane at night seen from a lighted room. When light is seen through darkness a colour arises which in this respect can be considered as the polar opposite of blue, i.e., yellow. Yellow arises when light is seen through darkness—e.g., a street lamp seen through fog, or a rising sun. As the light is more obscured by darkness, the yellow becomes orange or red, whilst blue darkens to violet. When blue and yellow mingle, green arises.

If we were to search through the history of art to find a painter whose work most livingly embodies the same realisation of the origin of colour as Goethe discovered scientifically, we come to one outstanding figure, about whom two very interesting points may be noticed, points which we shall afterwards see are intimately connected, although apparently unrelated.

Rembrandt was essentially an artist who stood as an observer of the real world around him, a somewhat detached observer, and the method of his observation was to see the deeds and sufferings of the world around him in a sea of colour arising from the interplay of light and darkness. Rembrandt's figures, homely and characteristic personalities as they are, are nevertheless even more essentially a part of the whole composition of light and darkness out of which they only partially emerge. Rembrandt sees his figures as part of a tremendous dramatic weaving and conflict between waves of light and waves of darkness. The colours arise out of the waves of light and darkness and the figures rise out of the colour—or, as in the case of his etchings, directly out of the light and darkness itself. Rembrandt is deeply concerned with the elements of light and darkness and everything in his paintings becomes subordinate to these, especially in his later works. On the other hand, another remarkable fact about Rembrandt in his earlier life was his fondness for painting portraits of himself. He made innumerable paintings, etchings and studies of himself, as though fascinated by the problem of self-realisation.

Let us turn now to what anthroposophy can tell us of the reality of colour as it flows through the living world of nature, weaving itself into the being of mineral, plant, animal and man, and find what correspondence there may be between this and the foregoing points of view exemplified by Goethe in science and Rembrandt in art.

In a lecture entitled 'The Creative World of Colour', Rudolf Steiner speaks of the living connection of a flowing spiritual sea of colour, with the colours of creatures and objects manifested in the external world. He says, for example, that the animal world lives wholly within the flowing sea of colour, and the fact that certain animals have skins or feathers of a particular colour is connected with the whole relationship existing between the souls of these animals and the whole (astral) flowing sea of colour. The animal is receptive in its soul to the colour which surrounds it and this flows through into the physical body. The polar bear, for example 'whitens' itself in response to its environment.

But man, in developing himself beyond the astral, or universal nature, to individual Ego-hood, lifted his head, as it were, above the flowing sea of colour and gazed upon it; and in gazing, he drank it into himself, and developed, instead of a colourful skin or bright-hued feathers and wings, a coloured, illumined, inner world of consciousness, of longings, of hopes, of passionate impulses, of aspirations, of courage, patience, inner strength. All that manifests itself in the outerworld of animal-forms and

16

colours—the white-hued, broad-winged gulls skimming the waves, the tawny, mighty-chested lion, the little darting lizards, green and brown, the patient burden-bearing grey ass, the great grey, burden-bearing elephants—all of these outer forms and colours find a correspondence in man's inner world.

Man has lifted himself above the flowing sea of colour; he has not taken it into his outer-being—the colour of his skin and hair—for had he done so, he would be like the animals, an unconscious participator in the work of the divine beings. No: man, as it were, has taken himself outside it all and surveys it; and in the surveying, he builds for himself, at first unconsciously, a living inner world.

The age when this inner world began to be lifted into the sphere of consciousness and of thought—the age of the spiritual or consciousness soul—corresponds with the age when first Rembrandt—intuitively as artist—and later on Goethe—more consciously as artist-scientist—advanced beyond the penetration of individual phenomena, of absorption in the particular, to a perception of the universal weaving of light and darkness through the whole visible world. They saw the living world of colour arising out of a sea of waves of light and darkness. They saw the interplay of these waves of light and darkness giving rise to colour. They saw the individual forms arising and expressed, each in their own quite different ways, the relation which they felt to exist between the whole sphere of light and darkness and the individual phenomena.

Rembrandt also expressed his self-consciousness, the consciousness of his separate, individual being, by first studying himself objectively in many portraits, and then with a certain wholeness of vision turned to the study of phenomena of the outer world bathed in a sea of light and darkness, out of which human feeling, human personalities, arose in colour.

There was a time when man, like the animals of today, lived in a sea of colour, and experienced it even in his physical being. Rudolf Steiner describes this when he speaks of the Ancient

Moon condition of our Earth. In the Earth period proper, man was destined to rise out of this condition to experience of his individuality, his Ego-being.

But whilst man, by developing his ego, has lifted himself above the animal forms which are the expression of the astral nature, his task now is, out of the consciousness gained in his spiritual, ego-nature, to turn again and spiritualise that in himself which he has surmounted but not yet transformed— i.e., to spiritualise his astral body. And as he begins to do this he will be led like a diver swimming open-eyed under water, to plunge again into the sea of colour from which he has emerged, and to take it, not into his physical body like the animals, nor merely into his unconscious life of feeling as at present, but into his conscious intelligence.

In so doing, colour will become alive and will speak to him— speak to him out of the green of the grass, the yellow flowers of springtime, the red and orange flowers of the summer, the mauves of autumn. The colours of the birds will speak to him, and not only their songs and cries. 'Nature, red in tooth and claw' will cry out to him its tragic tale of dumb suffering, and he will find a new pathway to understanding and sympathy opening up to him through the gateway of colour. A language is written in the world of nature around him, a secret language waiting for him to decipher, a language in which the mysteries of creation begin to be revealed.

In the red blood of the animal and man, and the green of the living plant-world, we have a pictured contrast which may lead us into a living relation with these two colours.

According to Goethe, yellow arises when light is seen through darkness, blue arises when darkness is seen through light, green arises when yellow and blue are so mixed together that neither in the least predominates over the other and green brings a feeling of satisfaction, of contentment. As Goethe says of green: '*Man kann nicht weiter, und man will nicht weiter*'

18

(you cannot go on, and you do not want to go on). It is a condition of absolute balance, of stillness and of rest.

But red has a very different character. Goethe says: 'If we intensify yellow we come through orange to red, and if we intensify blue we come through purple to red; so that red in a sense contains the essence or power of all colours—of the polar opposites of blue and yellow, and of all the intermediate colours.'

Rudolf Steiner says of red: 'Red is the gleam of the living, and green is the lifeless image of the living. For example, if we look at a red object, and then look quickly away, a green reflection or image is left on the retina.' Red shines into us and leaves us its lifeless image, green. 'Red, if approached through feeling, indicates something rather positive and aggressive.' And then in a wonderful passage he describes what may be experienced if we give ourselves up to the experience of red. He says:

> If we really unite ourselves with this colour we shall be able to have the following experience: I am here in the world. I have myself become wholly colour in this world: the inner being of my soul has become wholly colour. Wherever I go in the world, I go as a soul saturated with red, I live in red, with red, and out of red.

We shall not, however, be able to experience this in our more intensive life of soul unless the corresponding sensation passes over into a *moral* experience, a genuine moral experience. If, so to say, we floated through the world as red—if our 'self', and the world too, seemed wholly red, we could not but feel as though the whole world, together with our own being, were saturated with the substance of the *Divine Wrath*, streaming to us from all sides because of all the possibilities of sin and evil within us. We should feel ourselves within the infinite redness of space as before a kind of *Divine Tribunal* and our moral perception would become a moral perception of ourselves in the infinity of space. And if then a reaction comes ... it can only be what I might put into the words: *one learns to pray*.

With those two conceptions of stillness, neutrality and rest in the green, and of an almost awesome power in the red, we can begin to approach the worlds of plant and animal with a new understanding. In the wonderful beauty and harmony of the green plant-life which the Earth puts forth in springtime, we can feel what Rudolf Steiner describes as 'the Earth dreaming in the plants' – a kind of pure, delicate passionless imagery. In the passion-filled life of want and suffering of the beasts of prey and their victims, we feel the continuous urge and power living in red, manifesting itself in blind unconscious striving.

Red attacks us, overcomes us with a sense of its awful magnificence; it repels and fascinates. But when we can take it with courage into our being, ally ourselves with it and transform it inwardly, then the red blood of passion may become like the red rose in purity, like a fragrant breath of the World-Soul redeemed.

YELLOW

Let us now try to enter into the 'mood' of yellow in order to discover if, in its spiritual character, it can in any way be regarded as an antithesis to blue—as when regarded physically, it undoubtedly is.

Yellow gives a sense of joyousness. A field of daffodils or of buttercups gives a feeling of inward satisfaction, a kind of inward joyful strength. Just as the golden radiance of sunshine lights up the whole world for us, so yellow shines for us and gives an inward feeling of radiance. And because of this shining, radiant quality, the raying-out like sunlight, yellow is entirely robbed of its own nature if we try to confine it within definite borders.

Rudolf Steiner says: 'If we circumscribe yellow it is as though we were to mock at the essential *being* of yellow. Yellow will not be circumscribed; it wants to ray out on all sides. The old masters felt this radiant quality so strongly that when they wished to confine yellow within bounds they weighted it with metal-gold.'

And so whereas we give ourselves up in selfless surrender to the universe in blue, in yellow we experience ourselves in an inner radiant strength. A centre is created from which light rays forth continually into darkness. Such is the inward experience in the soul.

So in the worlds of plant and mineral, yellow gives us the feeling that some of the sunlight has been caught into the material and is doing its best to radiate still as a sun-reflection. Indeed the sun-drenched colours of autumn, when leaves and fruit turn golden, are nothing other than this.

In the life of soul, yellow is equivalent to the sunlike radiance of the spirit, brightening and strengthening the inner life.

Goethe says of yellow: 'Yellow in its greatest purity, always has the nature of brightness and clearness and possesses a serenely cheerful, gentle, charming quality. So on the contrary, it is extremely susceptible, and has a very unpleasant effect when it is a little dirty or to a certain extent thrown over into minus. The colour of sulphur, which tends to greenness, has something unpleasant in it.'

How do the dirty colours come about? As painters, if we enter into the life and mood of each colour individually, we feel a kind of love and understanding of it which helps us to bring it consciously into a right relation with other colours without sacrificing anything of its original character. If we are without such a feeling or conscious understanding of colour, we have either to cling to the imitation of nature, where the colour harmonies are already created for us to a certain extent in a sense-perceptible image, or, in abandoning this support to experience some uncertainty. Unclearness in thought and feeling about colour reflect themselves in the colour itself and dirty colours result. Yellow, red and blue in a clear relation create the

21

rainbow; in an unclear relation they neutralize each other and become a muddy brown or grey. A clear grey or brown can also be necessary as contrast, but yellow becomes unpleasant when a grey element darkens it to a greenish hue; red may be clear and radiant or unclear and darkened to a muddy brown, blue can become a dirty grey. In grey and black we have the image of dying and death. These are realities of the soul-life not only for the painter, but for everyone. Such thoughts prompt a question. What is it in our souls that allows us to accept the greyness of our modern urban world, without protest, and almost without consciousness?

Everywhere on the surface of the natural world, of plant and animal, there is colour and the language of colour speaking to the soul of man out of the soul of the Earth; everywhere where the intellectual striving of man has been directed through the mineral kingdom to a mastery of the sub-earthly forces of nature, to the mechanization of life, there the outward picture which results has been like a layer of greyness laid over the coloured Earth—in the form of our paved and tarred streets, grey buildings and the smoke pall that hides the sun. The greyness extends even to our physical organs. The human eyes which have in reality *a living power* of giving to their surroundings and are not merely a passive camera, become deadened by the greyness. By poring over newspapers, columns of figures and printed type, instead of reaching out actively into the blue of heaven, the power of physical sight begins to fade. The awareness of colour in the outer world has been a gift of the gods, needing thousands of years for its evolution. Man will lose this divine heritage unless he consciously wakens his soul to a more living relation with colour.

Greyness in the outer world means that the soul is being inwardly starved through lack of spiritual nourishment. Greyness in the inner being means that the soul is unable to create out of its own resources. A uniform greyness in the physical world would be a spiritual picture of approaching death.

22

In the world conception of ancient Persia, two spiritual beings stood in opposition to one another: the Spirit of Light and the Spirit of Darkness—Ahura Mazdao and Ahriman. The one was recognised as belonging to the forces of the Sun, the other as belonging to the forces within the Earth.

The conflict between the forces of light and darkness were conceived as a conflict between Ahura Mazdao and Ahriman for the rulership of the Earth. Anthroposophy teaches us that the same great spiritual being who was looked up to by the ancient Persians as the bearer of the sun-forces to Earth was He who later appeared and incarnated in the body of Jesus of Nazareth as the Christ who was the Light of the World. Ahriman—the Spirit of Darkness in Ancient Persia—is that spiritual being who in his legitmate sphere brings about death in the physical world, but who chains man's thoughts to the material world, to the Earth and to the sub-earthly, and who opposes the spiritual power of the Christ in mankind by exceeding his legitimate sphere and bringing about not only a physical death, which should release the soul and spirit, but a second death to the spiritual worlds.

Oppressed by anxiety or fear, or merely by the greyness of the physical world and atmosphere of daily life, the soul may, to begin with, tend to express itself in painting muddy unclear colours which are however a true picture of the inner condition.

With increasing consciousness, with a more vividly awakening power to live in colour, we develop the power of bringing light into darkness in the life of soul, to enrich it with colour. For the soul lives so intimately in colour that not only is a picture of the soul thrown out, as it were, upon the paper in painting, but there too it can be harmonized, balanced, made strong and clear and the clearness, radiance and harmony of the colours on the paper will react upon the health and clarity of the soul itself.

Yellow expresses a sunlike radiance. We should feel how the light is shining through darkness, how the power of the radiance of the spirit lives in yellow, dispelling the darkening forces of anxiety and fear in shining strength and courage. We may carry the power of red into yellow, and red is now no longer terrifying and overpowering but leads us to the elements of intensified spiritual courage in orange. The orange intensifies to a fearless yellow-red to vermilion, and there we have the characteristic colour of Mars.

PEACH-BLOSSOM

When, like Goethe, we look through the prism at a white line on a black ground, the rainbow colours appear. The white line is then entirely changed into colour: red, orange and yellow coming from above, and then green, light blue, dark blue and violet below. These are the same colours as seen in the rainbow and in the same order, but seen through the prism they have a dazzling intensity. They are the seven colours of the spectrum as generally recognised. Changing the white line on black for a black line on a white ground, we find a different group of colours. Here the darkness is in the centre, and the first image seen will probably be that of a dark purple, shading above through deep blue to turquoise, and below through red and orange to yellow. By changing the angle of the prism slightly we narrow the image; yellow and turquoise grow stronger, the purple narrower till at length the purple darkness entirely disappears, leaving only glowing pink-magenta colour which we name 'peach-blossom'. It is difficult to find anything more nearly corresponding to it in nature. The best example is the colour in the glowing cheek of a very young [white] child. The prismatic image is now yellow, peach-blossom and turquoise, not the rainbow colour range, but a kind of invisible completion of this, or, as we may call it, the other side of the rainbow.

Thus a new colour appears when darkness is transformed to light. The dark line disappears and a glowing peach-blossom takes its place. It is the colour of resurrection.

In such ways the colour-scale becomes living, the language of colour becomes intelligible and light and darkness, colour and the negation of colour, bring their spiritual message.

As the soul of man lives in colour, so the soul of the world lives in colour – in the coloured world of nature. As man pictures the life of his soul and of the soul of mankind in his creations in painting, so he also reads into the soul of nature by perceiving its life in colour, and he himself is bound up with it in its development. Colour arises between light and darkness, between the light of spiritual life and the utter darkness of spiritual death. Between earthly darkness and divine-spiritual light is set the 'Rainbow of Promise'. Man may feel cut off from the spiritual world, but he is never forgotten and the pathway of return is open to him.

If, as artists, we bring light into darkness we are creating in picture form a world of colour, and through our colour-imagination we transform the world about us.

If as human souls struggling through moral sickness and perplexity, we can bring light into darkness, we can begin to recreate in clear radiance the life of feeling and thought, and bring it to inward health—light bestowing. For whatsoever light we have within us shines outwardly. 'The Light of the body is the eye', and it is a light which gives radiance without as well as within.

The greyness of the mechanised industrial world around us may be taken into our souls; consciously or unconsciously it must be so in this age if we are to lead a full human life and not withdraw to a hermit's vantage. It is taken as darkness into our souls—but it must not remain so.

It is the task of present-day humanity consciously to permeate the darkness and transform it, to weave light into the darkness and transform it to colour, to bring life and light into a dying world out of the radiance of spiritual light and knowledge, out of an understanding of what was accomplished for mankind once and for all in the Mystery of Golgotha. And then, very dimly at first, we begin to realize more concretely the significance of the words of the Gospel of St. John:

> In Him was Life; and the Life was the Light of men.
> And the Light shineth in the darkness; and the darkness comprehended it not.

PART TWO

COLOUR AND HEALING

What is colour? What has it to do with healing? These are the questions about which an attempt will be made to find appropriate answers.

The answers should be significant. For whilst colour is becoming increasingly a part of modern consciousness, in art, clothing, interior decoration, and in healing, there are as yet few of us who are quite clearly aware of what colour really is.

This is not surprising since the theory of colour developed by Sir Isaac Newton in the seventeenth century, has been the foundation of our education and thoughts about colour ever since. Through this Newtonian theory, colour has been relegated to a secondary place in our scientific picture of the universe, whilst in our visual experience it creates the strongest impressions. So we have an anomalous situation.

We live in a coloured world, respond to colours in our emotions, use colours consciously to enhance these emotional responses, and create our own colours and colour moods within our own soul life. We even use colours physically in colour therapy, either to work through the soul upon the organs or even directly upon the physical organs themselves.

Yet do we know what colour really is? Though we may heal with coloured rays, the process is largely empirical and not clearly understood. A theory of split-up light, and of vibrations of varying speeds, increasing to unthinkable rates of wave movement, does nothing to help us to decorate our houses suitably with colour, nor to paint pictures with coloured pigments. This is a theory which we must and do learn to cheerfully disregard in practice.

Yet without this theory, we may be left stumbling entirely in the dark about colour, guided only by likes and dislikes. We may go forward using feeling alone, as do most painters for their incommunicable colour sense. Or we may, with Turner, take up Goethe's colour theory, and there find more satisfying explanations of the phenomena observed, a more accurate examination of the part played by the beholder himself, in his colour impressions.

Or again, we may leave colour aside as something intangible, and only of secondary importance to life, only waking to a faint uneasiness when we hear of an increasing prevalence of colour-blindness in our contemporaries. Not to know anything about colour may also have its dangers.

Yet colour, if it awakes in us lively sense-impressions, can work on us strongly. It can become the gateway to new worlds of experience wherein thinking and feeling together play their part. Let me recall a personal experience of this kind, strong enough to remain undimmed in memory over thirty years.

I stood, with others, on a little ridge between two groups of mountains. The sky was filled with wet tawny yellow vapour, as the last rumbling of thunder was dying away to the east, where a brilliant double rainbow arched itself high against the inky background of clouded hills. To the west the red disc of the sun was sinking below a range of mountains. When we turned to the left, there appeared to be a high arc of golden light extending from the sun to the rainbow. We turned to the right, and again, there appeared a similar arc of golden light. We gazed upwards and the heavens were filled with this mysterious red-gold glow. So far as the eye could see we were as though enclosed in a mighty bowl of golden moving coloured light, a bowl which had a double rainbow rim.

It was an experience of awe and splendour. Here were we, insignificant specks in a vast cosmic drama of light and colour, yet in some sense also its creators. For the rainbow appeared just there where it was, the arcs of golden light just there where they were, only for our eyes. For someone else at a distance from ourselves, the focus would change according to their position between the sun and the darkness. We were the centre of this appearance. And to left and to right the light took on the form of an arc because our eyes could see it only in that way. We were the centre of all the glory our eyes revealed; tiny beings enveloped in a world of splendour, which nevertheless revolved around us as its centre. What had we as human beings to do with all this magnificence which awoke in us only wonder?

I knew most of the answers as taught in the textbooks derived from the Newtonian theories, but they did not satisfy. Colour, we are told, is split-up light, molecules in motion, vibrations of varying speeds ranging from thousands of wavelengths per second, to billions and trillions, in the so-called ether. What had speed to do with the emotional experience of colour?

Further we learn that colour can not be said to have any real objective existence. So and so many wavelengths impacting the eye produce the sensation yellow. Who shall say where yellow exists — in the eye, in the wavelengths, or somewhere else?

Colour is also, we are told, a secondary quality of objects. How it is attached to the objects is unclear. The observer reacts emotionally to colour but why he does so is also unclear, since all that is established is the speed of the vibrations or waves connected with the phenomena of colours. So we are no nearer to any satisfying answers.

The double rainbow faded and the green wooded hills shone wetly in the splendour of the dying sun. Colour glowed from the luscious green of vegetation to the rose-tinted air, to the green-blue sky, and the scurrying clouds, now crimson. So my questioning on the nature of colour faded with the sunset to the dark night of speculation on which the stars looked down.

31

There is a peculiar significance about the asking of questions. Galileo and the swinging lamp, Newton and the falling apple, are symptoms of the spirit of enquiry which possesses the man of the fifteenth to the twentieth century for his further evolution. Equally significant is the direction of the enquiry, as also the moment of time in which a particular question is first asked.

There are instances in ancient mythology which illustrate this point vividly, notably the legend of Parsifal. For failing to ask the right question at a particular moment, Parsifal was thrust out of the castle of the Grail, and had to wander for seven years acquiring wisdom through bitter experience before he was again allowed to enter.

After his period of trial, by asking the right question, he acquired the power to heal the wounded king, Amfortas, and to become himself ruler of the castle. The legend has grown out of an ancient wisdom concerning the spiritual evolution of man. The picture it contains could be equally applied to our own times.

For the castle, symbolizing the head of man, contains his human intelligence, in which all sorts of questions arise at different levels, with differing aims. We have asked more questions in the last five centuries about the phenomena of the earth, than were asked in that direction in the preceding millennium. Nonetheless we have by no means exhausted the questions which may be asked.

Through not asking the right questions now about colour, mankind may find itself thrust out of its castle of the Grail, For colour is the earthly key to a portal of the worlds of soul and spirit, of which modern man knows so little.

NEWTON'S COLOUR THEORY

Prior to the seventeenth century, colour was considered to be directly created through refraction by sunlight. In 1666, Newton

IRISH CANCER
SOCIETY
LIMERICK

DATE 21/05/2024 TUE TIME 13:47

BOOKS		€1.50
TOTAL		€1.50
CASH		€2.00
CHANGE		€0.50
CLERK 1	279898	00001

made his discovery by his use of a prism, that all the colours exist already in solar light, and can be separated from one another through refraction. This concept persists in the textbooks to our day.

Without using any prism it is easy to convince oneself of this theory by a familiar experience. We put a tumbler of water on to a white tablecloth where sunlight can catch the top of the glass and by refraction reflect on to the cloth, and we notice the rainbow colours appear. Colour is split-up light, we explain to ourselves.

Yet the colour only appears on the edge of the light where there is shade, not in the centre where the light is the strongest. If it is all contained in the strong solar rays, why does colour cling to the shadowed edges?

Another experiment we can easily make is to look through a prism, if we have one. If not, through a bit of glass from an old chandelier from a second-hand shop. With the prism at the right angle, e.g., level and horizontal to the eyes, we look at a sheet of white paper. First we see only whiteness. Then colour — at the edges of the paper! Yellow, orange, red is above, and green-blue, blue, and violet below. They are just like the colours of the rainbow, but the green is missing, and there is a wide space of whiteness between. The colours again appear only where the whiteness meets the darkness beyond the paper.

Let us go a little further, and put a brushful of black water-colour paint on to the white paper. Look again through the prism. Colour leaps into view: yellow, turquoise, peach-blossom, magenta, violet. The most brilliant ones appear just where the darkness is strongest. It almost seems as though we could just as legitimately say that colour is split-up darkness. But what then of Newton's theory? Let us ask the physicists.

Professor Arthur Eddington answers this question for us. In a chapter entitled 'Discovery or Manufacture', in his *Philosophy of Physical Science*, he suggests that the direction of the thinking of the scientists may influence the results of their experiments.

In relation to the colours in the solar rays, and the theory arising from Newton's experiments, he says:

> The mistake was not in saying that a green component already exists in the sunlight, for that is, at any rate, a legitimate form of thinking, but in claiming that we could decide experimentally between two equally permissible forms of description. And by our oversight, it happened that the form of description we condemned was rather more natural and appropriate than the one we undertook to defend.

This puts the matter very moderately. Goethe felt much more strongly about it when he remarked to Eckermann: 'An error in thinking can lead centuries astray.'

GOETHE'S THEORY OF COLOUR

As Goethe gave the first importance to his Colour Theory, and much time and thought to exposing Newton's error, as he thought, in this field we can hardly doubt that he had this particular error in mind. Goethe could well understand that the way we put our questions influences the form of answer we obtain. He believed that Newton and his followers had erred because they put the question wrongly; and not this question alone, but many more, whose effects are experienced to our day.

The idea which was held by thinkers before Newton was that the light creates the colours by refraction. This seems consistent with our experience of colour as the most fluctuating and impermanent of all phenomena our senses perceive. Colour comes into being in the flowers, flourishes and fades. It plays over the earth and heavens in the sunset and sunrise; it glows transiently in the rainbow. Except in the metals, it has always the character of impermanence.

Newton reflected the spirit of his time when he looked to colours as something permanently contained in the light, e.g., encased in every ray of sunlight. To him, colour was not part of a process of creation, but each colour was an already existent entity — a permanent reality.

Goethe saw colours arising through a process of lightening and darkening: the darkness of infinite space seen through the light-filled air creates the blueness, likewise the darkness of distant mountains; whilst light struggling through a darkening medium, of clouds, dust or fog, creates the ragged orange of the storm, the yellow of a street lamp, the deep red of sunset. He saw the creating of colour as a living process, not a separating out of something pre-existing, but an active interplay of light and darkness, continually creative.

These three distinct concepts of colour seem to be related to the times in which they were thought.

When men thought of the universe as the work of a Divine Creator, the concept of colour and beauty as a continuous revealing of the creative process, was a natural one.

When the marvellous discoveries of physical science seemed to be showing material causes for everything, it was easy to form the concept of colour as a material something imprisoned in sunlight, and from thence to be separated out.

Goethe, however, was ahead of his time in discovering his idea of colours created by lightening and darkening. He knew, from inner awareness, that the colours had a spiritual significance which was being overlooked. He believed that the questions of the physicists were all being put in a way biased towards materialism and that many such errors would result. His view of colours was only one of the many scientific concepts in which Goethe in the nineteenth century was a forerunner of Rudolf Steiner's spiritual science in the twentieth.

What then is the way to put the question about colour in our own times?

We do not really believe any longer in the theory of the split-up rays of light. Neither, if we understand Prof. Eddington rightly, do the physicists. He describes how a demonstration of the theory might be staged to convince an incredulous 'spiritualist', and how it would fail. 'Yet', he writes, 'I think it not unlikely that even an expert might fall into this trap today — such is the glamour of an historic experiment. He really knows better; but one does not always recall one's knowledge when it is wanted.'

It may be inconvenient for the physicist to frame his questions in a new way. Goethe's form of questioning was only understood by the rarest souls amongst his contemporaries, and is only now beginning to awaken general interest. But humanity cannot wait for the physicists. We need to know the truth about colour, for colour goes far beyond physical science.

THE REALITY OF DARKNESS

One difficulty we have immediately to face. If colour is created by an active interworking of light and darkness, we can no longer regard darkness as a nullity. Darkness must itself be an active force.

For Goethe, as a Rosicrucian, this was no unthinkable proposition. But to his contemporaries, as to many Western thinkers of today, it seemed nonsense. Darkness is thought to be only absence of light.

It is, of course, peculiarly Western thought which denies reality to darkness. To Eastern philosophies, Yin and Yang, Ahura Mazdao and Ahriman, had equal and polar reality.

We shall try, in a later chapter, to show how the reality of Darkness as an active force may be justified even in our own experience. Darkness can be active spiritually in the souls of living people. Since Hitler, few will deny this. We have lost our nineteenth century equanimity about soul-darkness, and the active power of evil.

In such ways the understanding of colour leads on of itself towards a healing reconciliation between the two worlds in which man functions, the world of sense phenomena and the worlds of soul and spirit. For if Darkness is active, so also is Light. The Light of the World illumines the conscious human spirit.

Just as an unbalance in the human being to either side, the physical or the spiritual, a leaning too much to either sphere of experience, can precipitate illness, so an equilibrium maintained in the soul between the two spheres equates the poise of health.

Because colour is perceptible to the outer senses and also to the inner senses it is a borderland reality, true and perceptible in both worlds, therefore invaluable for the healing of both soul and body.

To reach to clear perception of colour in an inward way necessitates a way of self-development for which our age is ready, but as yet unaccustomed to pursue.

To realize the intimate connection between physical sight and the inner activity of the soul is yet another step in consciousness.

Further still is the realizing of colour as an active power in healing, not only in the physical treatments of Colour Therapy, but in a more psychological and spiritual way, as direct tonic, or curative treatment of the stresses of the soul.

The way to such development is open to the person of today. The condition of the world about us cries out for a spiritual science, an initiation knowledge, of which a true experience of the nature of colour may well become a first and most significant step.

COLOUR IN EVERYDAY LIFE

If we put out of our minds all theories or preconceptions of vibrations, wavelengths and the like in connection with colour, what do we know of colour through the evidence of our own physical senses?

Let us give a simple example of how colour speaks in ordinary life.

THE EFFECT OF GREEN AND RED

I travel by car along a country road through leafy woods clothed in the pale shimmering green of spring. There is a light rustling sound of wind among the branches, a light radiance in the opening buds, and the greenness conveys a feeling of cool contentment and promise of new life. On the road ahead of us is a red country bus, flaunting its utility. By the roadside we meet first a red postbox, and later a telephone kiosk, both drawing attention to themselves through their redness. Then we spy two ladies crossing the road clad in crimson coats, and a child wearing a beret of flaming vermilion. These also do not wish to pass unnoticed.

An artist painting the woods would seize on the vermilion beret or the crimson coats as a touch of contrasting colour to enliven the green. He would probably prefer either to the red bus or the red telephone box, unless he were a modern cubist painter. But he would not choose the ladies primarily for their personal charms, but for the enlivenment of a landscape through figures and for the way in which red enlivens green.

In such ways the painter lives into the language of colour, as a matter of the technique of his profession. We all do something similar, but a little less consciously. And not all painters are very colour conscious.

If we look on green, abundant as in the green fields in springtime, we can feel two things — there is life, and also a certain innocent tranquillity. The tranquillity belongs to the green. A green meadow, a green tree, or leafy forest, green coloured walls in interior decoration, or green silk hangings or dresses.

HOW WE REACT TO YELLOW

Quite different feelings are invoked if the green is shot through with yellow, different again if we have yellow itself, the bright yellow of spring daffodils or the golden yellow of a ripened cornfield, the flaming yellow of gorse, the pale yellow of a primrose bank, or the yellow radiance of sunset. There is an enhancement of life in the yellow, a joyousness; where the green leaves us tranquil, yellow shines like light itself. It would be difficult to sustain a melancholy mood in a room coloured yellow. Either the mood would succumb to the yellow and we should become gradually more cheerful, or, hugging the melancholy, we might feel inclined to leave the room — for the glow of yellow is consistently cheerful.

HOW BLUE AFFECTS US

Quite different again is the experience of the colour blue which we gain through our senses. Blue sky or blue sea or blue distance — all give a sense of spaciousness, something which draws us out of ourselves into a larger world. At its most intense, the blue of a summer midday sky gives us a feeling of dark immensity overreaching all pettiness.

Blue gives us the tranquillity of greatness, transcending small anxiety in an embracing peace. In its lighter hues, with white in it, blue has a gentle sportive cheerfulness, less active than the yellow.

These are all sensations we can have in looking at the colours, for which no theory is needed, only direct experience.

The colours convey themselves to us, too, with a kind of inner gesture. Yellow shines towards us, much as children experience it when they hold a yellow buttercup under one another's chins. It reflects like light, whilst blue has a constant elusiveness, a kind of mystery of withdrawal; it always moves further away so that one can never quite catch up with it. Whether it is the blue distance or the elusiveness of a bluebell wood, the blueness has a movement of withdrawal.

Red rushes at us like a fury, or flames sombrely or burns fiercely or with a fiery warmth, or glows with grandeur and power. It attacks rather than withdraws.

Thus each of the colours has some character of movement, but the movements are only qualities of the colour, not the colours themselves. The moods and movement of the colours give us the feeling that these have a direct effect upon us — they lure us out or drive us back or bring us to inner stability.

There is nothing in the wave-theory that explains such feelings. These are movements of a different kind, experienced qualitatively. They cannot be numbered or measured but are nonetheless real. We know this, through experience.

If one pursues this qualitative mode of thinking one can soon come to the idea that colour tells us something of the nature of a being, as the colour of a person's skin can tell us whether he is well or ill, or the colour of the leaves on a tree tell us the progress of the seasons. We accept the information given by the colour, perhaps without conscious reflection.

No amount of reflection would bring us to the idea that what we experience qualitatively is merely an increase or decrease in the speed of vibrations or wavelengths. This quantitative mode of thinking lies outside the contents of the sense perceptions.

Goethe's approach to knowledge was qualitative: his belief was that we should trust the senses as our means of knowledge, and not depart from them into speculative theories.

Yet even on the path of qualitative thinking we still must go further if we are to find out what colour really is.

ARE DREAMS COLOURED?

Another much more brilliant colour world opens for us when we fall asleep, and again not all people are conscious of it. One often hears or reads discussions about whether dreams are coloured. Some people, even some painters, assert that dreams are in monochrome, like a photograph.

In such a way might the physical world appear colourless to a colour-blind person. Such people are fortunately not sufficiently numerous at present to make us doubt the reality of colour in the outer world. It could come, but it has not reached that point yet. But we can lose the colours of the inner world. In this sphere we are more colour conscious as children than in later years.

I remember dreaming as a child of three great tawny yellow lions, in a sandy reddish desert, against a brilliant blue sky. Nothing could shake my certainty thereafter that dreams are coloured, until in later life this awareness of colour in dreams, awoke again. Yet our faculty for perceiving colours the moment our eyes are closed, dies, if it is not cherished.

The converse is also true. My students often tell me that their painting lessons start them dreaming in colour. It is not a new faculty of course, for we all dream in colour. We only fail to remember it clearly enough. One student who remembers having very clear colour experiences on the threshold of sleep as a child, lost these for very many years, and was delighted when they lighted up again through her work with me in painting.

Does this matter? It does matter because waking or sleeping, colour is the life of the soul. Our consciousness functions in two different spheres. But we are not two different beings, nor living in two separated worlds. Blindness to colour brings a dullness into the whole inner life, including the sleep life, for colour is the bridge we may most readily cross, from dawn-waking consciousness to the consciousness at present hidden from us, behind sleep and death.

Parallel to this, our senses wake up, and everything around us lights up in colour, when we begin to pay attention to colour in our waking hours.

If we could carry this awareness further to spiritual seership, we could be aware of a transformed and glowing world, scintillating and radiant in every leaf and flower. What we normally see is dulled by our own rather dull senses.

One might then expect that all painters would dream in colour. That very many do is evident through modern surrealist painters cultivating dream-consciousness as their inspiration. But the quality of their sleep or dream experience is influenced by the subjects they give attention to in waking life, be it form, colour, pattern, or dark and light.

The outer senses meet the inner, and what we take into the experiences of sleep is a kind of mesh of images mirrored into our consciousness through the day's, and behind that through our life's experiences. What we have experienced depends on how much the inner senses were awake.

The inner senses enliven the outer, and where one individual sees only a red postbox to remind him to post his letters, another sees how a red spot on the green background gives life to the greenness, a third sees how red rushes out from the greenness, and almost attacks one with its insistence.

Similarly, the dream-life of different individuals of a like sensibility may be prosaic and colourless, dramatic and colourful, or imaginative, vivid and significant.

The two kinds of experience of sleep and waking are only one and the same individual's life in its two aspects, and many a painter has not wholly escaped the darkened consciousness of his times, in seeing 'objects in space' blankly as pattern and form, rather than qualitatively, in colour and significance.

RUDOLF STEINER'S TEACHING ON COLOUR

The moods and movements of colour as described are not merely subjective impressions. Anyone can experience the same, if they approach colour in an unprejudiced way.

These impressions tell us something of the objective nature of colour, but to approach a qualitative science as Goethe tried to do we must bring the objective perception to the point of perceiving general laws. For this we may turn to Rudolf Steiner's lectures on Colour.*

These lectures were in a sense only the beginning of such a science. Yet since all Goethe's studies on the nature of colour were a foundation for Rudolf Steiner's further investigations, this beginning was an important piece of work. To give the contents of these lectures briefly is hardly possible, and it is only through working with the thoughts given in a practical way that the psychologist, painter or physicist can understand and appreciate them.

For whilst Goethe, working from an inner certainty of vision, tried to build up a physical science which included the eye which sees, and the various forms of colour appearance, both subjective and objective, Rudolf Steiner carried the study further still.

Having a clear perception of the soul world of colour, he showed the way to such an understanding of colour, through feelings, in what we may term the waking day-life of the soul.

Feelings have to be raised above the personal to the level of the super-personal, to objective general truths.

Can this be done? Rudolf Steiner said it can and must, if we are to understand colour. Those of us who work as artists with his indications, find them both true and helpful. But much more needs to be done in this direction.

Dr Steiner indicated how we can come to a closer understanding of colours and how to use them. He distinguished first between the colours in the sense of two kinds — lustre and image (*glanz und bild*), or the radiant active colours, and the colours that are not active in themselves but hold a given form. Thus red, blue and yellow are active lustre colours, green, peach-blossom, white and black are image colours.

It is not too difficult to follow him when he defines green as the image of life, peach-blossom as the image of the soul, white

* *Colour,* Rudolf Steiner Press, 2005.

as the image of the spirit, and black as the image of the lifeless. These definitions correspond with ordinary human feeling. But to carry these definitions further, as he does, is more difficult to follow, and for this we must turn to the lectures themselves.

In such ways we may come to objective laws of colour which experience can support. But through the images of life, soul, spirit and death we also come to the borderland of what the physical senses perceive. Beyond that borderland the rainbow hues of colour still beckon us on.

Is the real nature of colour beyond the senses' perceiving, or is it a call to awaken the senses to a more lively perceiving? Are we come to the point where colour is a gateway of the spirit, where the spirit through enlivened perceptions and thinking can cross the borders of the two worlds split apart at our birth?

If this is so, it will surely be comprehensible why Goethe, poet, philosopher, statesman and scientist, should, at the end of his life, say these words to Eckermann:

'As for what I have done as a poet, I take no pride in it whatever. Excellent poets have lived at the same time with myself, poets more excellent have lived before me, and others will come after me. But that in my country I am the only person who knows the truth in the difficult science of colours — of that, I say, I am not a little proud, and here I have a consciousness of a superiority to many.'

COLOUR, HEALING AND HEALTH

Colour is created by the light, irradiating the darkness.

Every night and every morning the mantling darkness meets the light, and the earth is transformed in a glory of colour. Every morning and every night, the light of the spiritual world meets and touches the fringe of our earthly darkened consciousness. The migrant soul is filled with colour, in dream, or in waking pictures.

44

Sickness nearly always betokens, in some sense, a rift between the earthly personality and its spiritual sources, between the incarnated soul and its discarnate spirit.

Many grave illnesses are preceded by severe depression; for example, an acute physical illness such as cancer, or an acute mental illness, of suicidal or homicidal nature.

In such illness there may be a kind of psychic darkness, experienced not only by the sufferers themselves, but even by the persons around them also. I can testify to this out of my own experience in healing, and I believe many people who have worked with mental patients will be able to support this statement. Something like a cloud of darkness, bringing acute depression, attacks one. The healer must be aware enough to confront it, otherwise he too could be overcome.

Many examples of this are too harrowing to relate. I have one patient in mind however who recovered, so far as I know, completely. A young man, he said to me once, despairingly, 'The world is growing grey for me. I long for colour, and can find no colour anywhere.'

Apparently, then he was in fairly good physical health, and I was puzzled. Actually he was on the edge of a complete mental breakdown which happened a month or two later.

MAN IS THREEFOLD

Just as we, as souls, live always in colour, between light and darkness, so do we also live, in feeling, between thought and will. As we are air-beings, when in our breathing we inhale and exhale rhythmically, so are we Light-beings, when the thinking we are unfolding is living in the light, yet do not know it, because we live within it.

In his lecture on 'Thought and Will', in the collection of lectures entitled *Colour*, Rudolf Steiner explains this contrast at some length. Thinking is living in the light, whilst Will is unconscious. Thus man can understand himself only if he takes himself as a seed of futurity, enclosed in the past, in the light-aura of thought. '... Light shines out of the past; darkness leads into the future. ... In Will is revealed finally the continually beginning, the continually germinating world.'

A healthy balance of thinking and will is maintained through feeling. In a like way, the balance is maintained physically between the head system and the metabolic or limb system, through the rhythmic interplay of blood circulation and breathing.

It requires a lively and imaginative power of thinking to enter into this concept of health as a mobile balance, between opposite kinds of forces. Yet it throws great light on the complex nature of the human being.

Our head and nerve-senses system is continually destroying nerve substance as we achieve consciousness. So the present age is 'nervy'. Too much activity in the head nature in early life, may result in thin spidery limbs; in later life, it may cause sclerosis: in thinking, it may produce an intellect without imagination and without feeling. For these conditions, art in education is a corrective.

The metabolic activity is continually up-building substance. If this becomes excessive it can produce corpulence, sluggish thinking and sometimes false growths, tumours, etc. A helpful corrective is to arouse enthusiasm in exercising the creative faculties in the arts.

A peculiar illness which occurs through an unbalance between the digestive and head nature, is called migraine. If we were clairvoyant we might lie down after a heavy lunch and see colours. The digestive system creates colours. This is a fact which might profitably be studied by the Surrealists.

In migraine, one is suffering from the digestive activity extending upwards into the head, and a symptom may be to see lights, or colours moving rhythmically in a blinding brilliance, which symptom often precedes sickness and headache. This illness is not generally well understood. My own impression is that it can be caused by meditation made too soon after a meal, so that forces are drawn too strongly into the head. I find that a strongly-willed meditation on one colour can banish the irregular many-coloured symptoms and avoid headache, if taken in time. Also there is a medicine which helps to restore balance between head and metabolism.

Polarities of head and metabolism should be balanced in health by the rhythmic system of blood and breath in the 'middle-man'. Because this system should be healer of the other two, illnesses which affect the breathing, such as asthma, or hysteria, are difficult to heal. These can be helped most through the arts; through colour, music, rhythmic movement and rhythmic occupations such as weaving in colours, or through rhythmic speech or breathing.

The soul has always to find and keep its balance between all these polarities; between head system and metabolism, between thinking and will, between light and darkness, between past and future. In all these, health is not a static, but a mobile condition of balance.

The soul that cannot find and keep its balance between all these polarities, finds illness instead; and out of illness may win the new consciousness that helps to re-establish its balance in health.

ILLNESS CAN BE A BLESSING

Illness is not necessarily a misfortune; it can be a great blessing. For through illness we may find ourselves able to take time to survey the whole of life and to realize more of its meaning and aims. Whereas the person who always enjoys 'rude health' may enjoy his body so much that he forgets the beginnings and ends of life; rather as a small boy, running an errand for his mother, may enjoy the diversions of the way so much that he forgets what he started out for. We are all rather like children in this respect; and illness may serve to remind us of our spiritual origin, otherwise too frequently forgotten.

The conflict between thinking and will, between light and darkness is familiar enough to us all. 'For what I would, that do I not, but what I hate, that do I.' The struggle between all these is the ego's effort for spiritual self-realization.

In black darkness we can do nothing. Darkness is hostile even to life. But light transforms darkness. In light, life thrives, and lifts itself up to its highest manifestation, in the consciousness of man.

How then do the colours bring healing?

The whole living world radiates colour. Though it is true a pale plant may be grown in a near dark cellar, its life will then be as frail as its colour. From the splendour of tropical flowers to the rosy bloom on an infant's cheek, the living world glows in colour endlessly. The colours fade in sickness and death, as the plant-world dies into carbon, or coal-blackness.

Colour can be stimulated within a living being, either from outside, or from inside. Colour healing which involves the use of coloured lamps, is principally concerned with treatments from outside. Other means we may now consider are concerned more with awakening an inner consciousness of colour.

COLOUR THERAPY

In the early part of this century Rudolf Steiner foretold that Colour Therapy would play a great part in the coming times. We are now seeing it used in different ways in colour treatments. Of these perhaps the most widely known are those which use coloured lamps for treatment of the patient externally through the skin, either directly on to affected parts, or through so called 'colour baths' where the patient is immersed in a space filled with and surrounded by one colour.

Most of this work is in a stage of immaturity which does not court publicity, but many beneficial results are claimed for healing inflammatory conditions, and treating sensitive conditions not responsive to other medical treatments. Rudolf

Steiner distinguished two kinds of colour treatment, one which acts directly upon the organs, and one which acts more through the organs of consciousness. The latter is the means generally employed in the clinics and curative homes which have developed out of the indications he gives. Here again, the treatments through colour are in process of development, and only a few indications can be given, though those interested could follow these up at the institutions mentioned. (Arlesheim Clinic, Switzerland; Sunfield Children's Homes, Clent; Rudolf Steiner Camphill Schools and others.)

COLOUR AND THE EYES

The use of colour naturally plays a considerable part in the treatment of the eyes. Colour treatments are more potent if contrast reactions are used. For example, red and blue may be used to correct short or long sight by a rhythmic succession of contrasting experiences of first one colour, then the other, ending with the one most needed.

Blue lures the vision outwards, and so helps short-sight; red drives us back into ourselves so can help to correct long-sight. Activity in the eye can be increased by a rhythmic and balanced alternation.

The use of colour is not confined to treatments of the eyes. It is still more potent in affecting consciousness. In the curative homes of the Camphill Community, colour is used in combination with music to affect the disordered or undeveloped soul condition of what are generally called children in need of special care.

The use of moving coloured shadows thrown on to a screen, in a room coloured appropriately and filled with string-music, can have a wonderfully healing effect on children and others suffering from cerebral palsy and other nervous conditions of our age, if it is used with an adequate artistry. One needs to become an artist in healing to use such methods effectively.

THE USE OF RED AND BLUE

Colours can be used to heal illness of either the upper or the lower organism, through concentrating the effects of red, or blue; through, for example, making one room entirely red, in walls and furnishings, and another entirely blue, and letting the patient experience the room alternately.

The isolated effect of one room or the other is less significant than the contrasting reactions through the rhythm changing. Blue walls deflect functional activity from the head to the rest of the organism. In a completely red room the effect is reversed.

Rudolf Steiner gave indications such as these, as to how colour may be used effectively in restoring a healthy balance in functional activities.

Experiences in colour therapy show that colour plays a part in our well-being, even in the physical organism.

Psychological treatments also reveal that a patient's illness may often be shown through his paintings, both in his choice of colours and of forms — in other words his illness reveals itself in his soul. The self which forms the mirror for our life's experience may get clouded or dull and the colours it reflects may take on a greyish hue.

Alternate red and blue treatments will not do much here, for the patient has now to take in hand the enlivening of his own soul life, through his own efforts, and to do so, there can be few things more helpful than painting, used not in a diagnostic, but a curative and ultimately an artistic way.

For the first step in healing is the inner effort of the self to hold itself erect in its environment. Through an awakened sense of colour, one begins to awaken to the world around us in a new way.

The soul lives and rejoices in colour. With awakened perception of the world around us we begin to respond livingly to the life around us revealed in a coloured world. Colour speaks to us, and our soul's response is a renewed joy in living.

Through painting, and all its aesthetic laws of colour harmony, balance, etc., we learn to balance ourselves. Through creating out of colour, we discover the inner creativity in ourselves; through discriminating selection and imagination, we learn to draw upon our senses' observations, our balanced judgment, and the limitless wealth of images which the world beyond dream supplies and find, out of our own sources, that we are creators.

In the physical space-world to which we have been rather closely tied during the past five or six centuries, painters have placed things side by side, or behind or before each other, conforming to the laws of space, where certainly two objects cannot occupy the same space at the same moment. Perspective has ordered these spatial arrangements for us by making the near things larger and the far things smaller, and so on.

But the soul sphere, behind the dream and behind the artist's imaginative faculty, has no such limitation; one object can appear out of another, like the genie out of Aladdin's lamp.

Colours are transparent and weave through each other like a luminous coloured smoke. Forms are not static, but in a constant process of change. Life weaves through everywhere, soul gleams through every colour. Spirit speaks through colour, movement, light.

COLOUR EXERCISES

Through colour exercises we can establish a healthy and harmonious balance in the soul.

Taking flowing water-colours, and making them flow freely on the paper as sunshine flows freely through the air, we do not at first need to think of depicting anything, but only of living into the mood and movements of the individual colours. So to spread outwards with the yellow and to feel a condensing and drawing together in the blue, can be like a soul exercise in inbreathing and outbreathing.

One can make pictures of moonlight or twilight, and find images out of the colours; or one can just paint for the enjoyment of the colours themselves.

It is effective because the soul's life is lived in colour, and it is good to remember now and then, in the hurly-burly of existence, that we each are possessors of a living soul.

We may paint with all the colours eventually but at first it is best to take them singly as a means of entering more deeply into their individual characters.

Each colour shades off into two others; e.g., yellow to greenish and orange-yellow, blue to purple and green blue; and so on. Each colour has its own character, e.g., orange gives courage, green gives tranquillity and balance, and so on. Each one provides a voyage of discovery in its many tones and nuances.

Or again one may stimulate each by the use of complementary or contrasting colours. A pair of complementary colours are a colour drama.

To find the complementary, one has only to paint a bright spot of colour on a white paper, gaze at it for say, twenty seconds, then transfer the gaze to another uncoloured paper, till the eye conjures up the appropriate complementary.

One can use colours in other ways than painting, without resort to a 'treatment'; coloured lights, coloured reading lamps or coloured hangings may help. I have one friend who found it impossible to sleep under an orange coloured eiderdown, but slept peacefully under a blue one. In regard to these things one must learn to use one's own discrimination.

Painting, however, has one great advantage. It builds independence in us. We are alone with ourselves and the colours. Nothing happens until we can take courage and begin.

We reveal our own emptiness or are astonished at the creative imagination we discover unexpectedly in ourselves. Either way it can be a wonderful path of self-discovery, and what is negative soon becomes positive, if we persist.

COLOUR AND THE FOUR TEMPERAMENTS

The individuality is the key, the one true Self finding its way between all the colour varieties of temperament — sanguine, melancholy, phlegmatic or choleric.

The sanguine temperament flits gaily like a butterfly from colour to colour, as from occupation to occupation in life, its illness is restlessness and indetermination.

The melancholic temperament enjoys sympathising with fellow-sufferers, and descends deeply into blue and violet.

The phlegmatic pursues an undisturbed slow course through life and his colours may be muddy and undistinguished, but not that nor anything else troubles him over-much.

The choleric seethes with energy, and rejoices in fiery red colours, unless, as sometimes happens his temperament goes too far even for himself to contend with.

For example, a lady who attended one of my lectures, stood up at the end and complained of my saying that colours were of spiritual origin. 'Look at red!' she declared. 'How can one say red has a spiritual origin? I loathe red!' One felt from her tone, that to her, red had something of the character of original sin.

I looked at the lady, and understood her trouble immediately. She was choleric to the verge of illness — absolutely bursting with redness, and this outburst was characteristic. She could not stand any more of red in her vicinity.

Paradoxically, in the treatments of the Rudolf Steiner Curative Homes for Children in Need of Special Care, an intensely choleric child is dressed in red with the purpose of exciting an opposite condition inwardly, by the re-action of the complementary colour, green or blue, to develop tranquillity.

In adults the colours seem to work differently. The soul seems to strive towards the colours it longs to acquire, but has not yet achieved, in its own aura.

The colour of clothing used to be a reflection of the aura. For a long time now it has been what fashion prescribes for us.

Coming generations will feel again for the colours which reflect the changing aura through life. We can all do this to some extent already.

Colours are the enliveners of both our inner world, and our outer world. They are objective realities, and individual necessities.

We cannot indicate a colour prescription for individual ills, for no two souls are alike, but with a few such indications as have been given, the individual can find his own colour. The finding will also be healing, for this will in itself be an individual spiritual deed.

COLOUR MEDITATIONS

Whenever we forget that we are primarily spiritual beings, we may easily let the affairs of everyday life overwhelm us with anxieties; we may fritter energy in over activity, in meaningless occupations, or get depressed because we are not achieving any spectacular success in any chosen direction. Disasters in the earthly life may overwhelm us.

At such times, when it is essential to realize the inner life of spirit, we may find it most difficult to sleep. As sleep is everyone's way into the life of the spiritual worlds, there is no better means of healing than first to re-establish the rhythm of sleep.

Colour therapists recommend a dark-blue lamp at the bedside to induce sleep. But if one takes instead the way of meditation, then one must know how to meditate. For meditation is intended to enhance consciousness, so that one can retain a certain awareness in that condition of sleep in which we normally have no awareness at all. For this kind of inner control and development of higher faculties we should refer to Rudolf Steiner's books *Knowledge of the Higher Worlds* and *Occult Science — an Outline*. Otherwise an attempt to meditate without guidance, might achieve the opposite effect from that intended.

All meditation must begin with an emptying of oneself from all outer sense impressions with the exception of the one chosen for the meditation. Take the colour blue. It is difficult to exclude unwanted thoughts and impressions, so to begin with one may use a memory picture. Remember as strongly as possible a blue sky, perhaps a night sky filled with stars. Or a blue sky over the sea where the blue is reflected in a myriad lapping waves, moving rhythmically. Or picture a blue cloak, and imagine oneself wrapped in it, so that the blue garment envelops eyes and ears.

There are two elements; the one the separating of oneself from unwanted thoughts, by holding one selected thought in the forefront of consciousness; the other, the blue, which has the character of lifting one's consciousness beyond earthly concerns to the awareness of the greater world which we experience in sleep. Insomnia is an earth-bound condition.

I remember a patient who suffered from sleeplessness, and told me that she had been dreaming that she was trying to get into the wrong house. This was an excellent illustration of what we all tend to do when we try to carry the concerns of waking life with us into sleep, instead of preparing ourselves, through thought, prayer, or meditation for the spiritual worlds we enter through sleep. To lift oneself to the immensity of the blue vault of heaven, in picture, can be a good preparation.

In a lecture by Rudolf Steiner in London, now published as a booklet entitled *Man as a Picture of the Living Spirit*, he gave a meditation which can lead us to some understanding of what is behind sleep. He referred to this meditation as one which reaches out to the true 'I'.

The meditation is as follows:

I gaze into the Darkness,
In it there arises Light —
Living Light!
Who is this Light in the Darkness?

55

It is I myself in my reality.
This reality of the 'I'.
Does not enter into my earthly life.
I am but a picture of it.
But I shall find it again.
When with goodwill for the Spirit
I shall have passed through the Gate of Death.

'Entering ever and again into a meditative saying of this kind,' said Rudolf Steiner, 'we can confront the Darkness. We realize that here on Earth we are only a picture of our true Being, that our true Being never comes down into the earthly life. Yet in the midst of the Darkness, through our good will towards the Spirit, a Light can dawn upon us, of which we may in truth confess: This Light am I myself in my reality.'

HOW TO USE COLOURS

Our world is beginning to rediscover colour.

After the drabness and sobriety of the nineteenth century, especially after the last decade of the twentieth, people awakened to a thirst for colour, in textiles, clothing, furnishing, advertising and illustrating as though in reaction to the bleak materialism of the preceding century, and to its aftermath in the horrors of war.

This path of discovery which was in a sense opened by Turner in the middle of the nineteenth century, has revealed itself in art, but not only amongst professional artists. Many brilliant amateurs have discovered that colour is an unending field of delight and discovery and are turning to painting for their own joy and satisfaction in middle and later years.

Amongst these one of the most notable of course is Sir Winston Churchill, who has enjoyed his terms out of office in the nation's affairs with great satisfaction in the study of painting. His delight in the colours is expressed characteristically:

'I cannot pretend to be impartial about the colours. I rejoice with the brilliant ones and am genuinely sorry for the poor brown ones. When I get to Heaven, I mean to spend a considerable time of the first million years in painting and so get to the bottom of the subject. But then I shall require a still gayer palette than I get here below. I expect orange and vermilion will be the darkest, dullest colours upon it and beyond them there will be a whole range of wonderful new colours which will delight the celestial eye.'

With his genius for language Sir Winston has chosen the right word. Only the celestial eye should be recognised as a possession, not simply in the years after death, but here and now.

If we would but learn to use it! Where man has adventured others may follow and, in so doing, discover something of the illuminating power of this celestial eye. G.W. Russell ('A.E.') has termed it 'The Candle of Vision'; it is in fact the eye of the spirit possessed in germ by us all.

A friend once came to see me in a depressed state of mind. She wore a dress whose utilitarian drabness revealed her inward condition.

Life had become a round of perpetual 'duties', whose performance gave small satisfaction to herself or to anyone else, but to which she was enchained by family conventions of behaviour. She felt it all foreign to her own real self, but had practically given up the struggle to assert herself, and was following a path of self-abnegation in a listless sort of way, which it seemed clear to me would only lead to illness.

I persuaded her to paint out of colour and followed this up by getting her to introduce colour into her garments. By the end of a couple of weeks she went home again in a greatly enlivened state of mind and the problems which had seemed insoluble were found to have partial solutions. She was able to satisfy her family's demands on her and still have opportunity for a creative and colourful life of her own.

This is one only of many examples of such cases of the revivifying effect of an enhanced awareness of colour.

The impact of the nineteenth century on our own times is perhaps felt most severely in the kind of education most of us have had, which has concentrated on developing the intellect at the expense of those higher creative facilities which can only be awakened and trained through the arts.

This is a deprivation which can hardly be overcome in one generation, since the teachers of the present generation still suffer from the utilitarian aims of their predecessors.

But it can gradually be overcome by many individual awakenings. The impulse to such awakening comes frequently out of illness, the cause of which it would hardly be too much to say is a starved soul-life due to our mis-education in respect of the arts.

BECOMING MORE ALIVE TO COLOUR

What everyone can do for himself to correct this condition is to become more alive to colour in his own immediate environment, both in nature and in the environment created by man of interior decoration, lighting, etc., and in his own clothing.

There are signs that men are awakening to the drabness of their city and business clothing. American men have revolted at the uniforms of utility and already wear colours that would seem daring in Britain. The Continent is more colourful in the surviving influence of peasant dress than our industrial population manages to be. But there are signs that men are beginning to resist the uniform sobriety which has been the outward and visible sign of their subjection to the task of making money, and are beginning to demand not only comfort but also some cheerful notes of colour in their clothing.

These instincts of revolt should be encouraged, for the age of drabness in clothing has been only a comparatively short one, which, if one studies the period, was almost equally drab in every other idea. It was the age in which agnosticism flourished;

an age in which the satisfactions of the material world were apparently sufficient to make the question of a future existence of no particular moment; it was an age in which men, women and children could be sacrificed on the Altar of Mammon, renamed human progress.

It is certainly not without significance that coincident with these ideals the business man has spread the blight of industrial smoke over the countryside and the drab uniform of servitude on his own person. It is a condition which is fortunately changing through many individual revolts.

As regards environmental conditions, the problem is rather more difficult. Our streets and houses may be painted more gaily; that change is coming, if not already here. But the problems of interior decoration are more intimately concerned with the soul-life of the individuals who spend their time inside the dwellings or work-places and here what is needed is a greater awareness of how colour speaks, below consciousness, to us all, so that colours can be chosen wisely.

PAINTING OUT OF COLOUR

There is one field in which every person is his own lord and master and that is in the field of his own creative activity. He may never have learned in the art-schools, nor in the ordinary schools, to draw and to paint, but that is no great hindrance.

WE CAN LEARN WITH GREAT JOY AND SATISFACTION TO LIVE WITH AND CREATE OUT OF A SEA OF FLOWING COLOURS. ANYONE CAN DO THIS.

All we need is courage, a pot of water and some brushes and tubes and then a sheet of white paper on which to begin to arrange this world of our own in which the colours shall flow, in which to do consciously in waking life what everyone of us does in sleep, e.g., to find the power of the creative self who lives in us behind our normal consciousness. It is not a plunge into a mystical heaven nor into a subconscious world of our own personal imaginings. But it is an honest effort to lift up into full consciousness that inner noble life of feeling and artistic sensibility which, as human beings, we all share and which only the dust of a century of materialism has overlaid. The sheet of white paper becomes for the time being the field of creative activity into which we each mirror our own soul's feelings and creative imagining.

What a plunge! Everyone shrinks back and says, 'Oh, but I am not at all gifted; I do not know how to begin.' This is really a shocking admission for it is an indictment of our whole culture.

Everyone knew how to paint when he was a little child. Every little child paints joyously still — why did we leave it with our childhood? Because we were led to believe that it did not matter very much. Machines and motor-cars drove out the colours.

But colours belong to the world from which we came, by which we live, and to which we shall return. The little ones know it because they have only recently left that world. We have so estranged ourselves that now we hardly dare enter. It is another world of experience but one that we need, most urgently, now!

Psychiatrists have discovered that by a process of 'doodling', or of letting hand and eye take their own path freely in black and white, or its equivalent in drawing and painting, they can encourage their patients to a kind of private confessional of their subconscious longings and desires. This can be helpful in diagnosis.

An inspector of education, in trying to discover the roots of a certain uneasiness she felt about present-day education, inspected herself, and came to the interesting discovery that there is hidden in us a creator who, given opportunity, is able to speak to us through the forms of art. In a book entitled intriguingly. *On Not Knowing How to Paint,* J. Field described her adventures in discovering this unsuspected creator in herself and how free paintings produce pictures of significance, not only of import for her own self-realization, but sometimes prophetic of future events, even of world events. Thus, free painting became for her a path of investigation of unknown forces and of a spiritual awareness hidden in the depths of the soul.

Something similar is indicated in J.W. Dunne's *Experiment with Time*. Here he recounts dreams where the future is forecast accurately twenty years before the event. These studies suggest that space-consciousness has been replaced by time-consciousness in the experience of dreams.

There are many further implications in this, of course, which we will not at this moment draw. (For further implications of this discovery see *Goethe's Conception of the World* by Rudolf Steiner.) Only the indication that within us, every one of us, is a hidden Creator and knower, who saves us from many foolish actions in moments of crisis, by a sudden 'hunch' but whom we effectively neglect in the larger part of our waking life in the pursuit of activities of seemingly more, but actually much less, importance for a full human life.

In *On Not Knowing How to Paint* the author stressed the hunger for she knew not what, which beset all her early artistic studies. Art, as it was taught in the art schools, did not satisfy. She could sketch a charming landscape but reviewed it without satisfaction. Less than the thing seen, it also did not satisfy that creator urge in her which was seeking satisfaction. Whilst the first incompetent free painting, which showed to her something unique and peculiar to her own inner striving being, was satisfying in its uniqueness and at the same time enticed her with its inadequacy to further and greater efforts. By these means a path was open, of which no man could tell the end, a path of self-discovery towards new world-discovery.

Modern Surrealist Art sometimes takes this direction but the results show it has some dangers. The colour world is the world of soul and there is a duality in the soul which reveals itself — as Goethe puts it:

> Two souls, alas! reside within my breast.
> And each withdraws from, and repels its brother,
> One with tenacious organs holds in love
> And clinging lust the world in its embraces:
> The other strongly sweeps, this dust above,
> Into the high ancestral spaces.

Not all revelation comes from above and painting that is swamped by the organic symbolism of dreams or the colours created by digestive activity may be interesting but can hardly be called art. This is the danger of the Freudian element in free painting, which can only be overcome by spiritual training and a growing awareness.

If one takes the path of objective colour study, something else enters from the outset. This world of colour is no private domain, filled with the demons or devas of the subconscious. Colour is that soul-element which we carry within us which rejoices with the coloured world around us.

We are living both in our own most lively creative power and in closest contact with the soul of nature when we rejoice in and create out of colours. We steep our senses in the blue of the heavens, the green of the earth, the scarlet, yellow, magenta and violet of the flowers; the crimson glory of the sunset. The universe speaks to us through its colours. We breathe them in through the senses. It is an in-breathing which brings life to the soul.

But there is also an out-breathing. The soul rejoices in colour and creates out of its own coloured world. We become painters, painting out of colour, whether of the visible world or of the invisible world — it matters little. As painters we must weave between these spheres just as in ordinary life we sleep and wake and carry our dreams into earthly creating.

So, from the visible world we draw forth the ideas which its forms reveal, not imitating but creating, whilst from the worlds invisible in which we experience behind sleep, we bring forth longing to unite this world of colour with our daily life in forms of beauty.

The soul-world, which was lost from sight at birth, begins to draw nearer to our consciousness. This is no subjective fantasy. Poets, mystics and artists from all time have known this 'many coloured world'. To awaken to it in our own consciousness is to bring strength, certainty and healing into the whole of life, for therein we all are rooted. (See *The Human Soul in Sleeping, Dreaming and Waking*, F.W. Zeylmans van Emmichoven, New Knowledge Books.)

How should one start then to paint out of colour? If one paints a landscape, does one merely imitate the landscape in front of one or does one paint one's idea of the landscape?

Is one a better painter if one paints every twig and blade of grass before one in realistic detail, as Ruskin would have us do, or if one paints a 'Nocturne in Blue' like Whistler, or draws a bull-fight like Picasso, full of whirling forms, bits of horses, bits of bull, bits of human forms in turbulent struggle. The nineteenth century loved Naturalism and the twentieth century seems to be striving to get at man's inner responses to the outer world. If one has seen a bull-fight, Picasso's drawings give a lively sense of the turmoil of feelings it excites. It is the 'idea' of a bull-fight — not the bull-fight itself. Turner did something similar with his landscapes. In his early years he made clever and exact representations, frequently nearly monochrome. At the end of his life he painted them as colour and idea.

What then, if we, starting with colour, as the subject of the painting, let it grow into expression of an idea? It may sound fantastic but there is a reality behind it, the reality of the 'many-coloured world'.

We belong to two worlds in our experience of waking and sleeping; in birth and in death we are as much at home in the one as in the other because it is only in our present stage of consciousness that they are two. In reality both worlds are one. 'As we are born into it, we split our world in two.' From then onward 'observation comes to us from the outside; the idea-world appears to us from the inner soul'. 'I look at the visible world; it is everywhere incomplete. I myself with my whole existence have arisen out of the world to which the visible world also belongs. Then I look into myself and see just what is lacking in the visible world. I have to join together through my own self what has been separated into two branches. I gain reality by working for it.'

The artist works or plays between the visible world and the many-coloured world, the world of the ideas seen by the inner eye. He is not deserting the visible world. He may be interpreting it, in terms of his inner experience, e.g., Picasso's bull-fights, or he may be shedding the glory of the 'many-coloured world' over our ordinary work-a-day one. But the seed of his imaginative creating is his own. It exists neither in the one world nor the other. It is a new creation coming into being. For the seed of the universe of the creative spirit of Man. In man is the Christ-seed of a new Creation.

Knowing this creative spirit exists in us, we can trustfully take the path through colour.

We learn to know the colours one by one — to radiate with yellow, to condense into form with blue, to glow with the warmth of red. We live with the movements of the colours — breathing outward with yellow, drawing inward with blue. We become pedantic with green and courageous with orange and vital with red.

But there is no short cut to discovery of the creator within us. We have each to discover it through our own effort, and colour is only one of the many paths to the spirit.